People Perish for a Lack of Knowledge: Self-Assessment

by Dr. Michelle McGrone

Publisher: Dr. Michelle McGrone

www.facebook.com/platediagnosisdoctor

www.facebook.com/thinking4lifeshow

Cover by Dr. Michelle McGrone

ISBN: 9781691046379

People Perish for a Lack of Knowledge:

Body Assessment

<h1 style="text-align:center">About the Author</h1>

Michelle has a love for technology and health. Dr. McGrone's educational background in technology consists of her Bachelor's of Information Technology (B.I.T.) with a specialization in Computer Forensics. In that program, Michelle graduated with high honors as Magna Cum Laude with a 3.84 G.P.A. and inducted into the International Honor Society for Technology Professionals (Epsilon Pi Tau of Delta Delta Chapter). She went on to her Master's program of Information Technology with a specialization in

Information Assurance and Security (M.I.T.) graduating with a 3.83 G.P.A. Upon completion of her graduate degree, Michelle went on to her doctoral program of Business Administration with a specialization in Computer and Information Security, passed all four comprehensive examinations on the first try, and began her dissertation on Advanced Biometric Technology, Non-Invasive Electro-Encephalography, and Remote Neural Monitoring more so on continuous authentication of human subjects and the prevention of hacking.

Dr. McGrone has practiced holistic healing for over 30 years. Ms. McGrone is known as the Plate Diagnosis Doctor. As the Plate Diagnosis Doctor, Michelle simplifies the basic mechanics of holistic healing. Her

greatest joy comes from teaching and guiding others with

the knowledge to heal themselves (to be a fisher of men

of their health and healing). Some of the teachings are

from first-hand knowledge as she becomes the study

subject of research.

 *Print is larger to accommodate vision impaired

individuals.

Table of Contents

Introduction

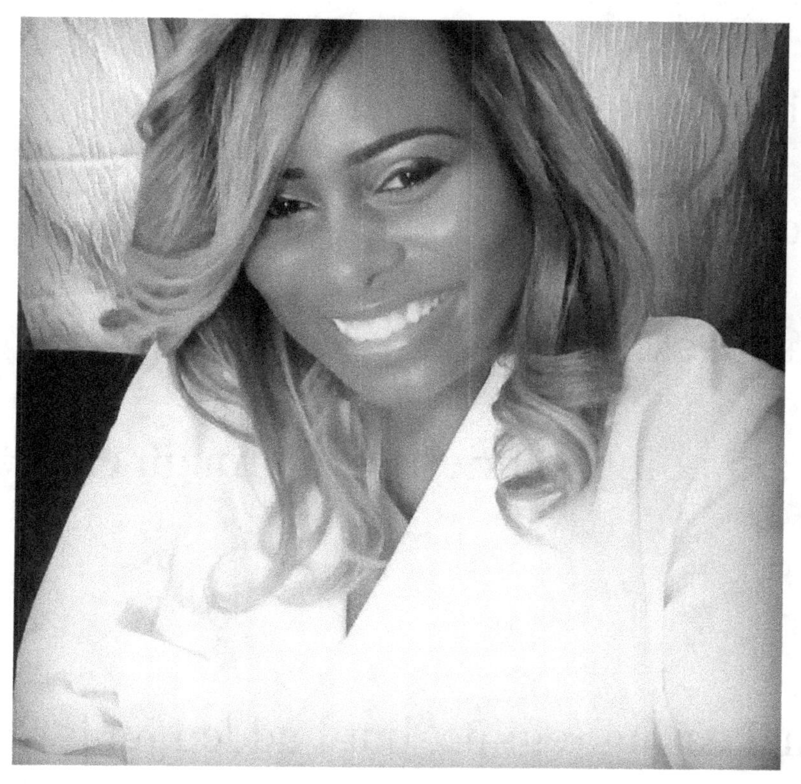

In the previous book the topic was on self- assessment. This book is on my self-assessment and discovery. For many years, I have practiced health and holistic healing. However, it was secondhand/secondary information. So, I decided to get firsthand knowledge by taking myself on a year-long study to gather some information. What I discovered was amazing. I discovered that there is one common denominator to sickness and disease when it comes to eating food. I will talk about each discovery in separate books. The focus of this book is to share my self-discovery results: head, hair, skin, eyes, tongue, lips, chest, stomach, fingers, back, knees, feet, internal organs, and overall feeling. I am going to briefly go through each result per body part.

I started my normal eating regime, but I added junk and fast foods and cold liquids (no alcohol consumption).

Head

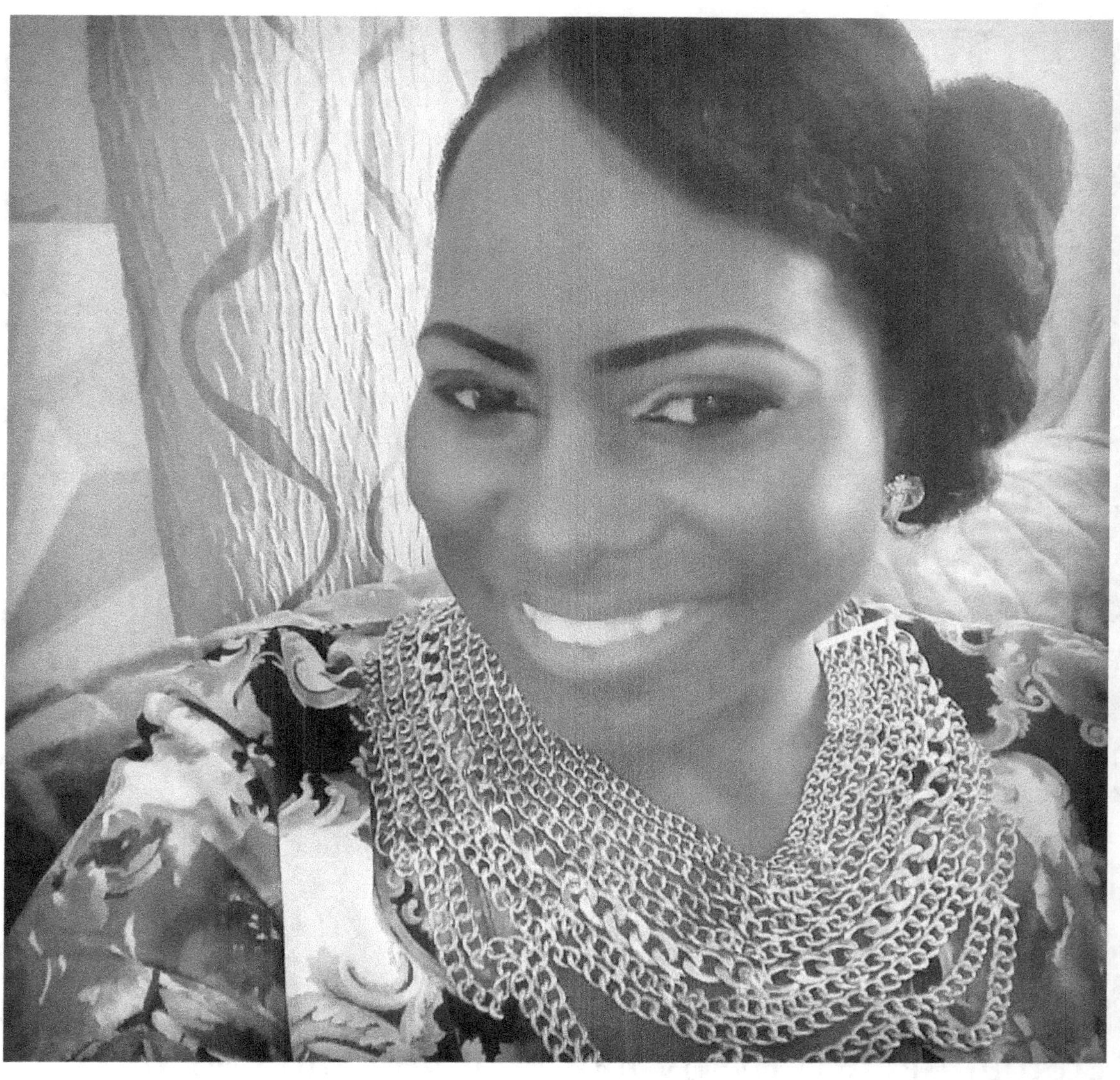

I noticed that I was easily distracted, my mental clarity was dull, more agitated, less patient, and headaches (Normally, I do not have headaches.)

Hair

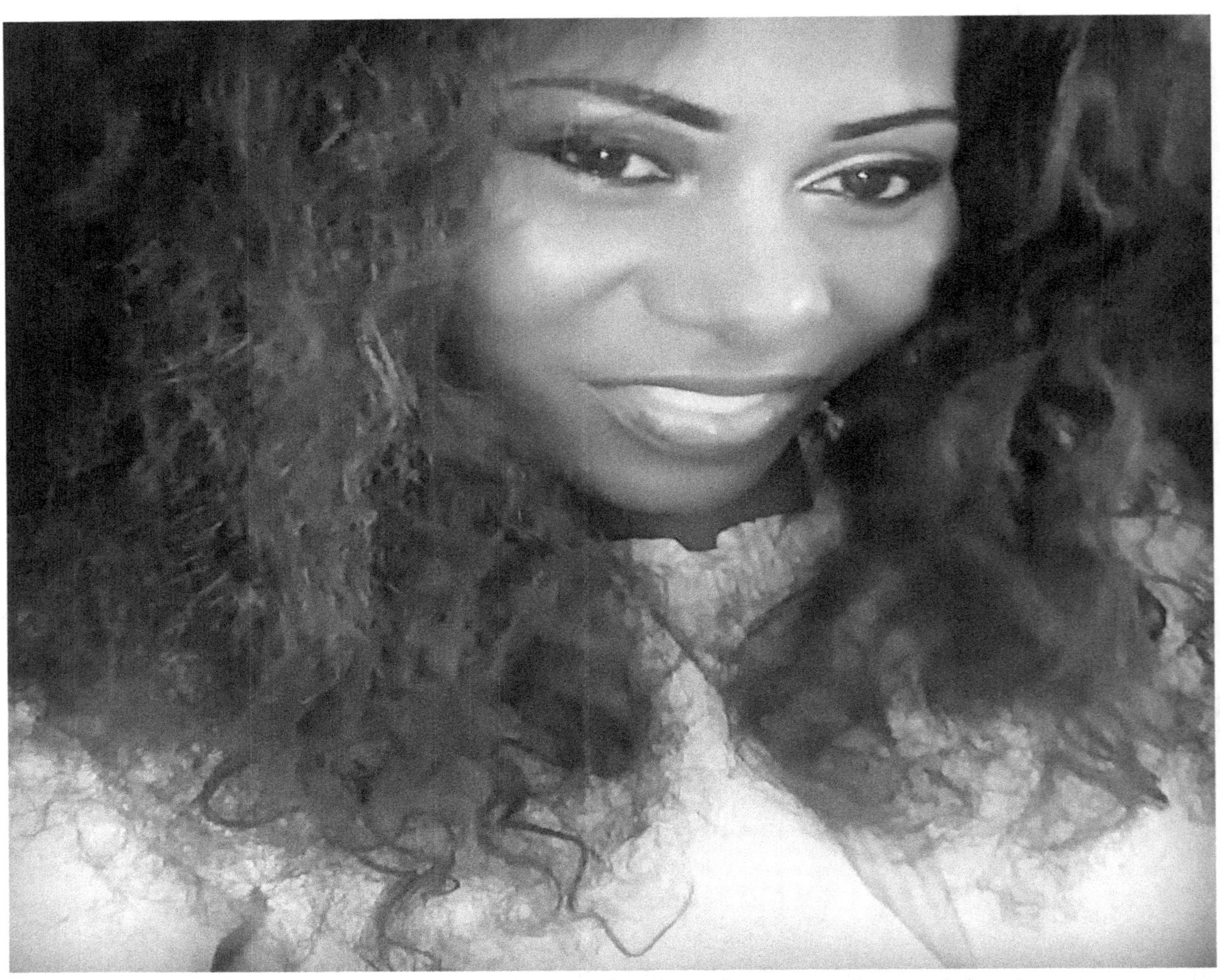

I noticed that the text of my hair changed and became more coarse, thinner, and dull.

Skin

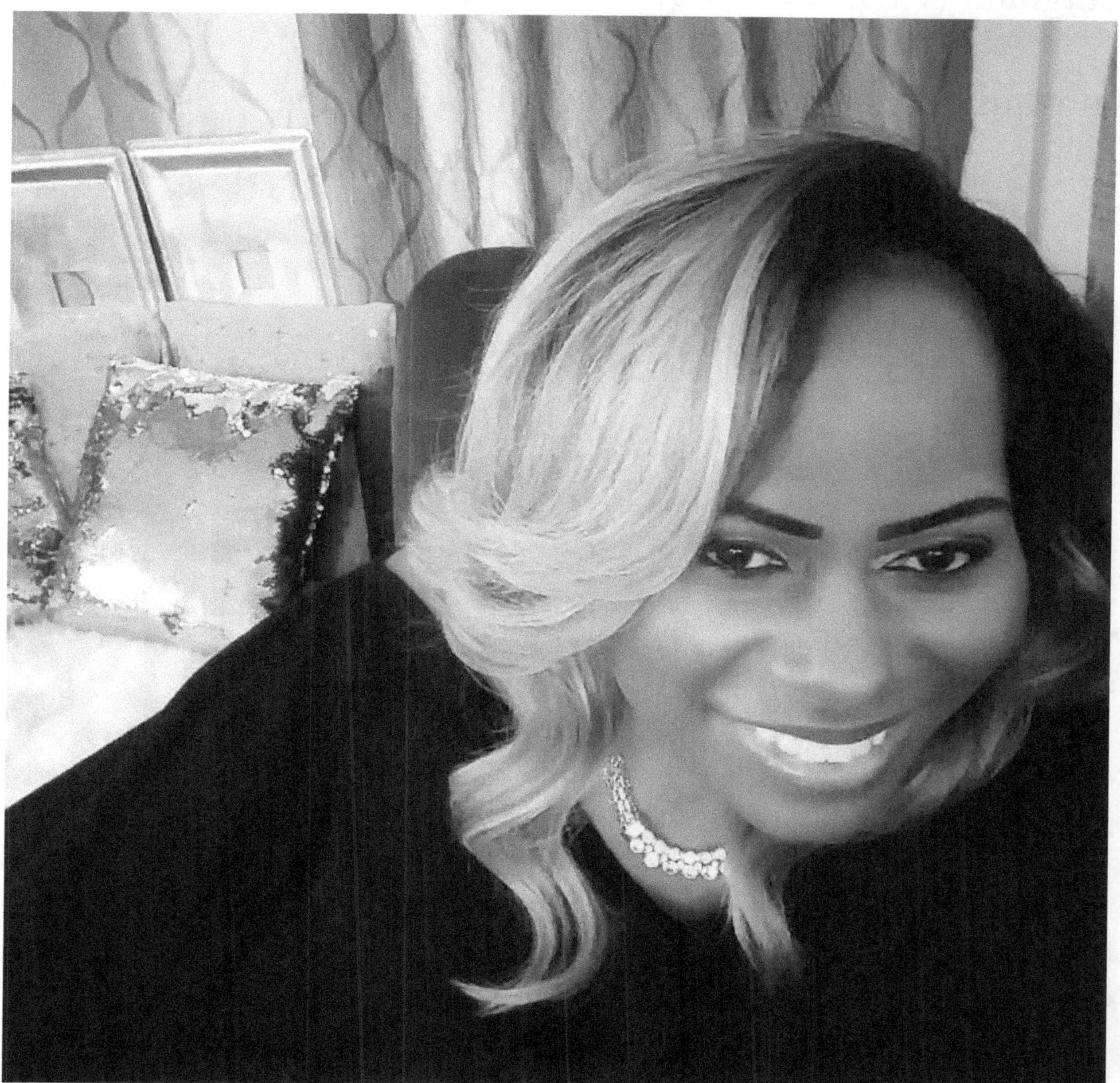

My skin became dryer and itchy. I also noticed that I was

being bit by lots of mosquitoes, too. I believe that when

you eat lots of foods that causes your body to become

stagnant (I will talk about this in another book.), it attracts

mosquitoes to you.

Eyes

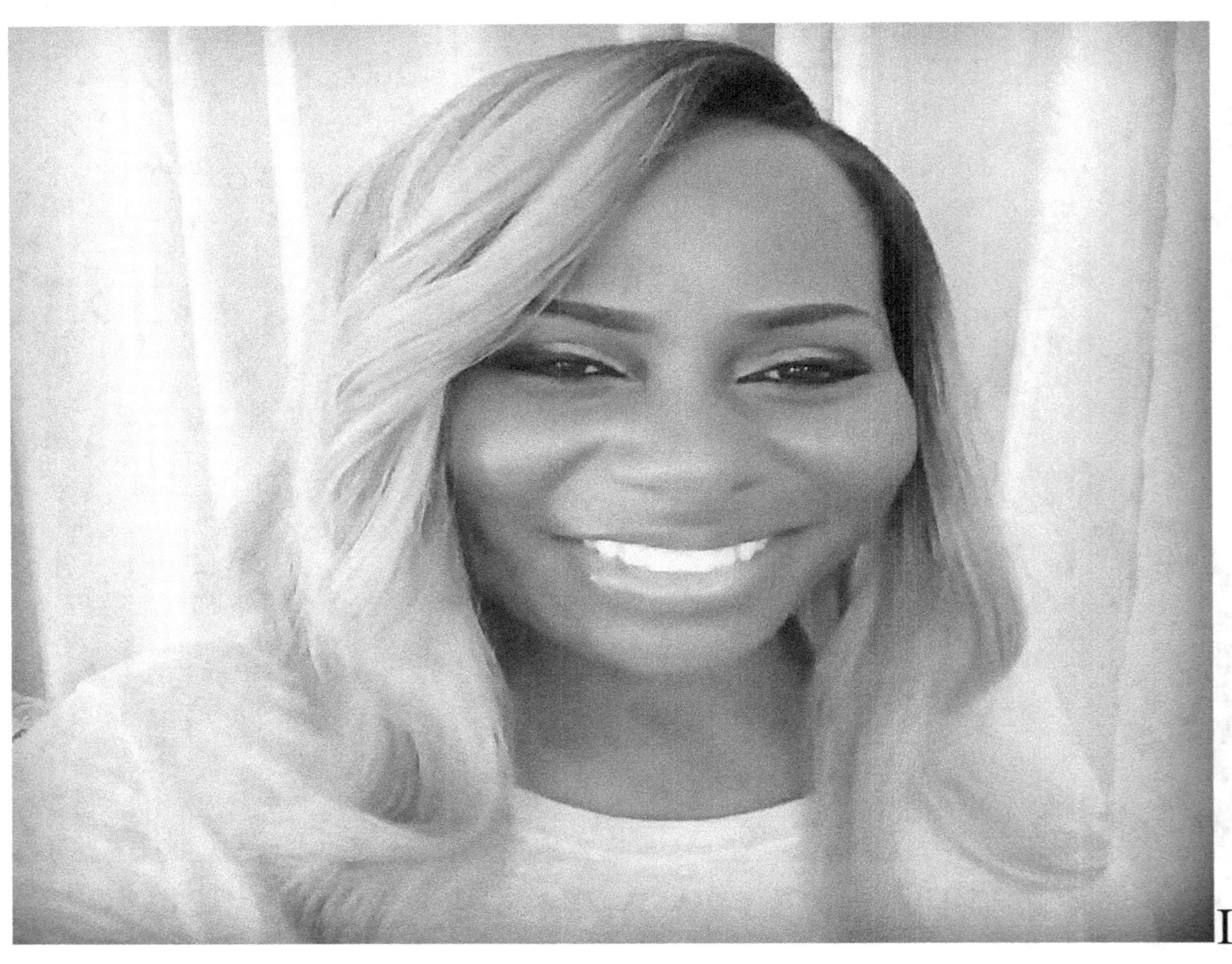

noticed that my eyes became less white and slightly

yellow, and sometimes my vision was blurred.

Tongue

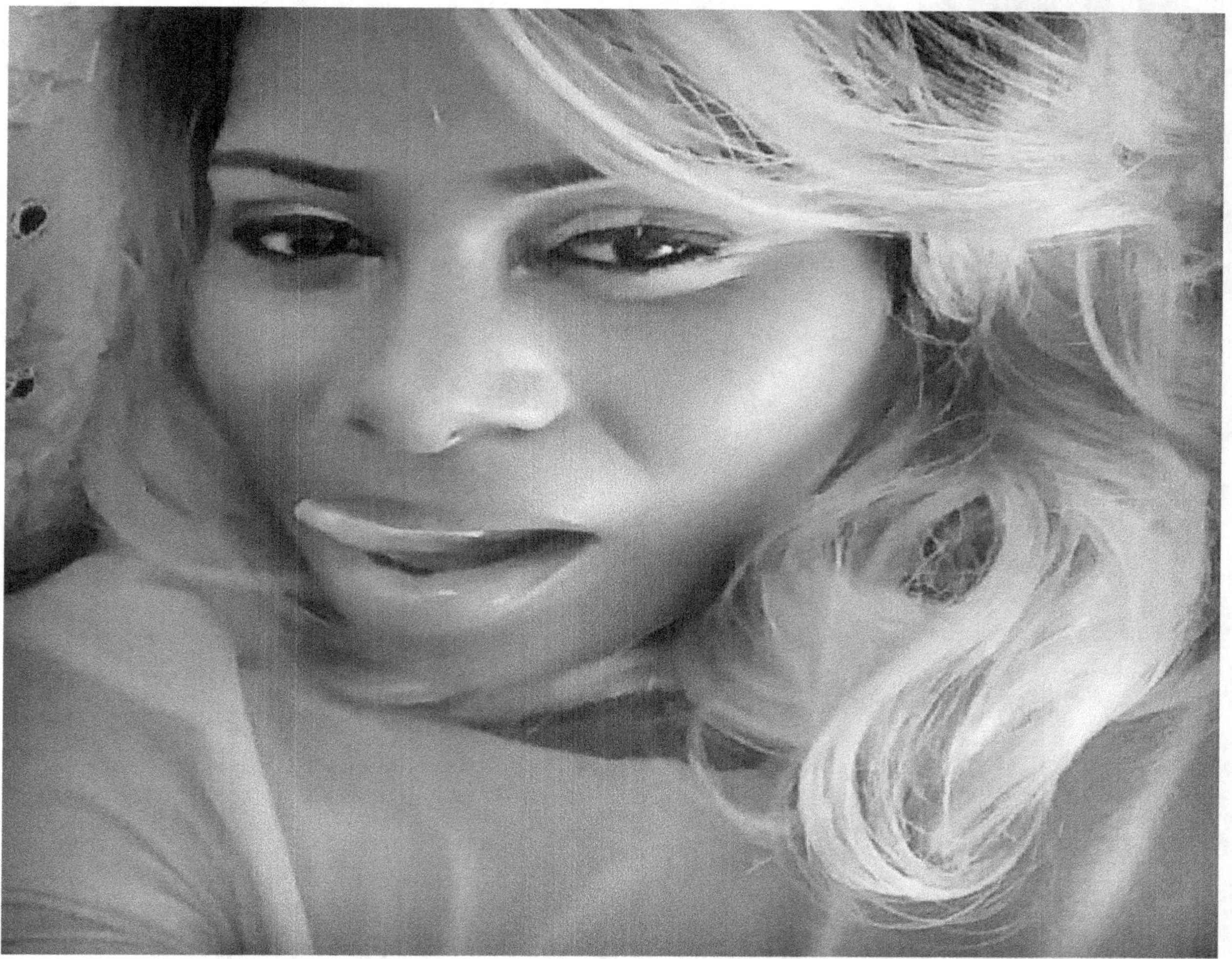

I noticed that my tongue was collecting and storing yeast

and becoming paler.

Lips

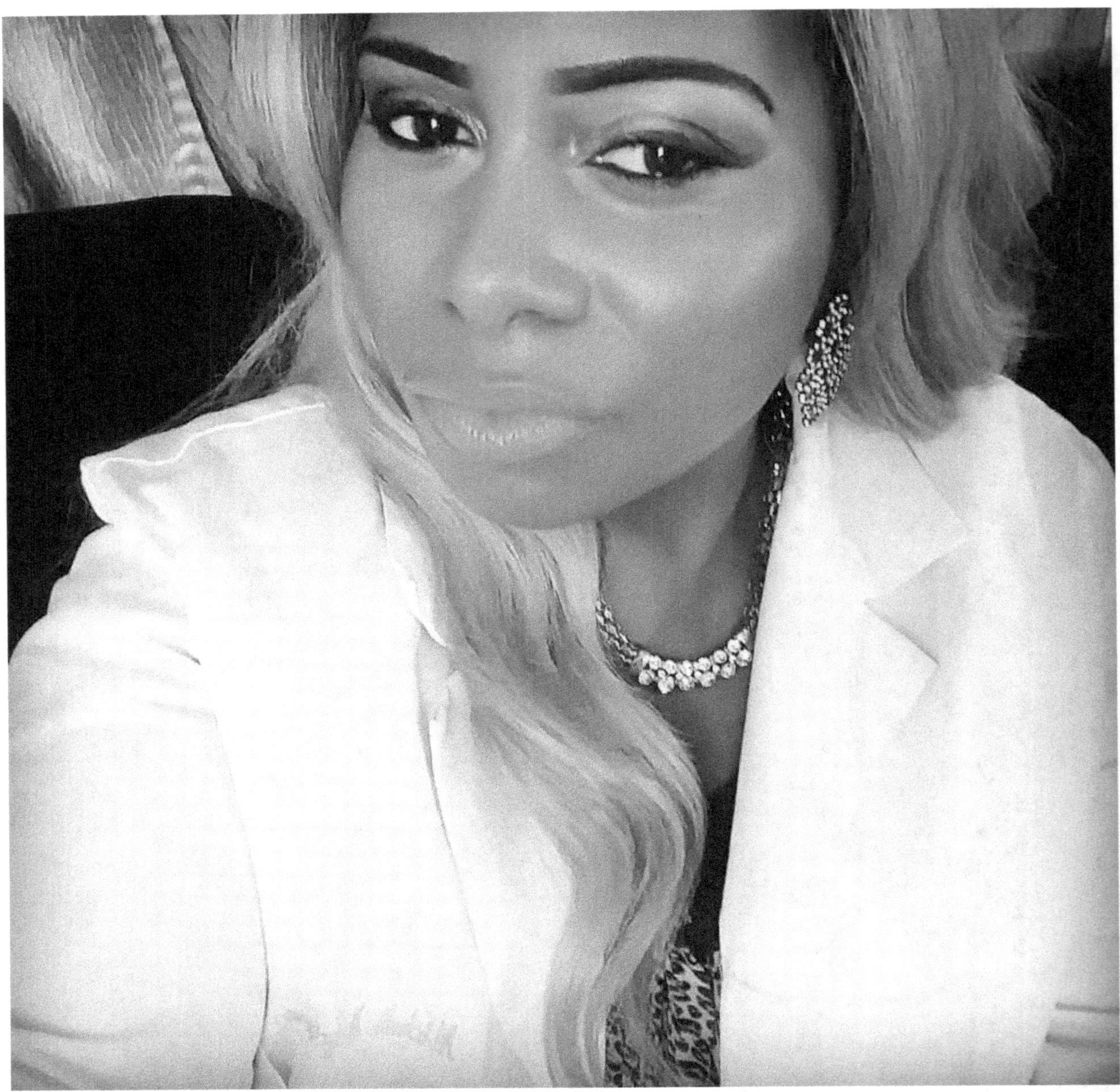

My lips were changing colors, were dryer, cracking, and sometimes twitching/spasms.

Chest

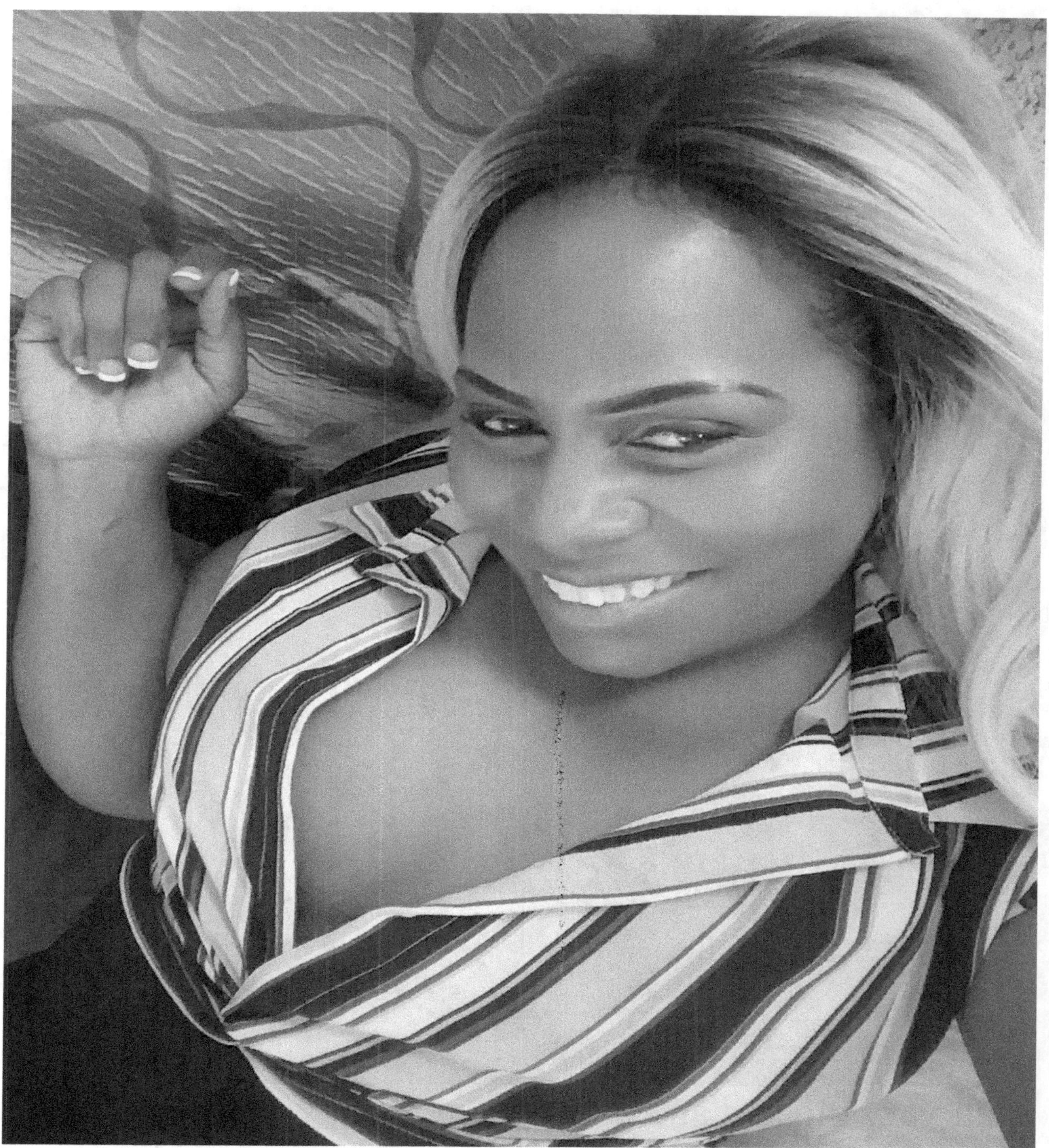

I started noticing tightness in my chest.

Stomach

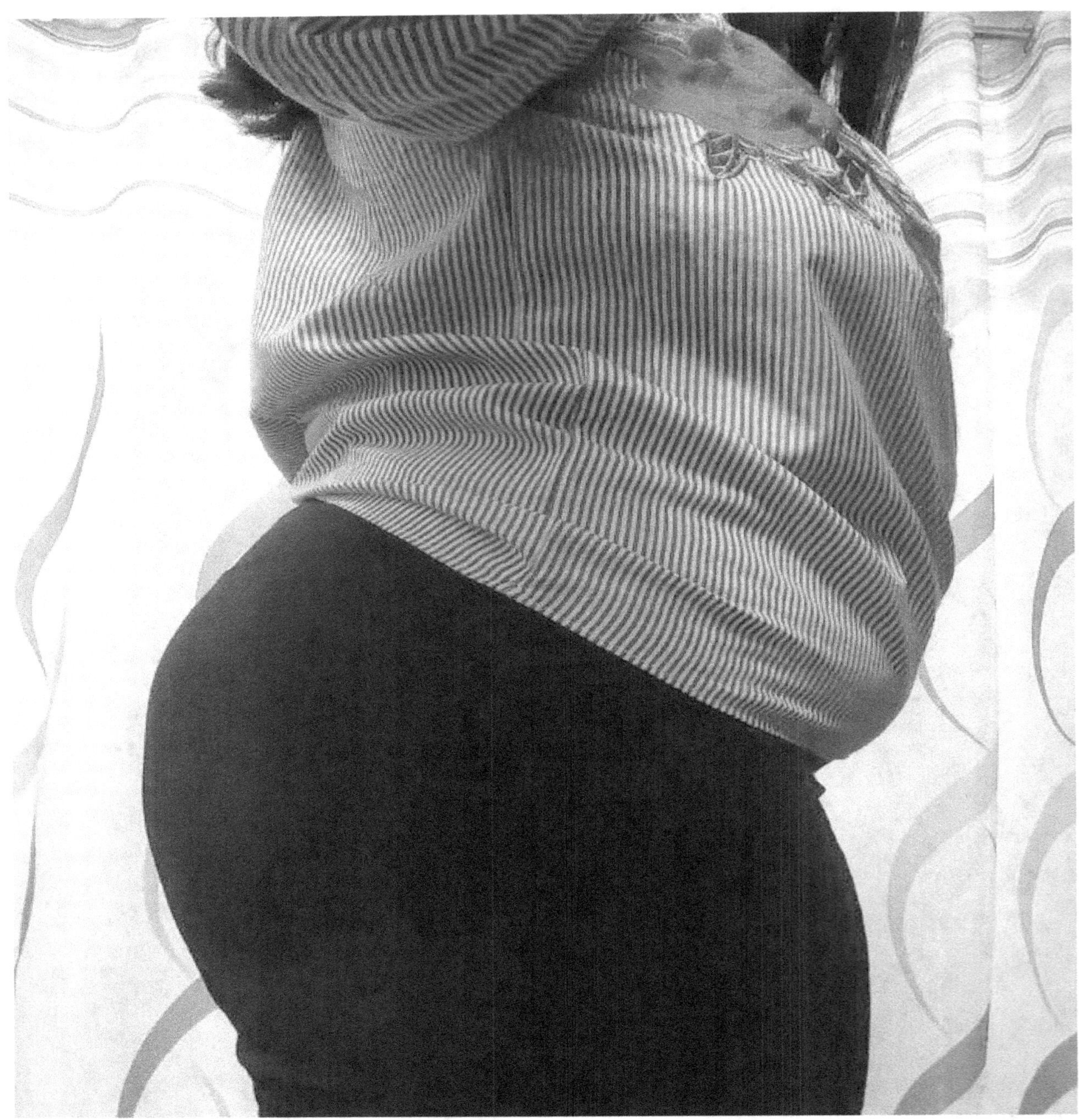

I felt very bloated and constipated.

Fingers

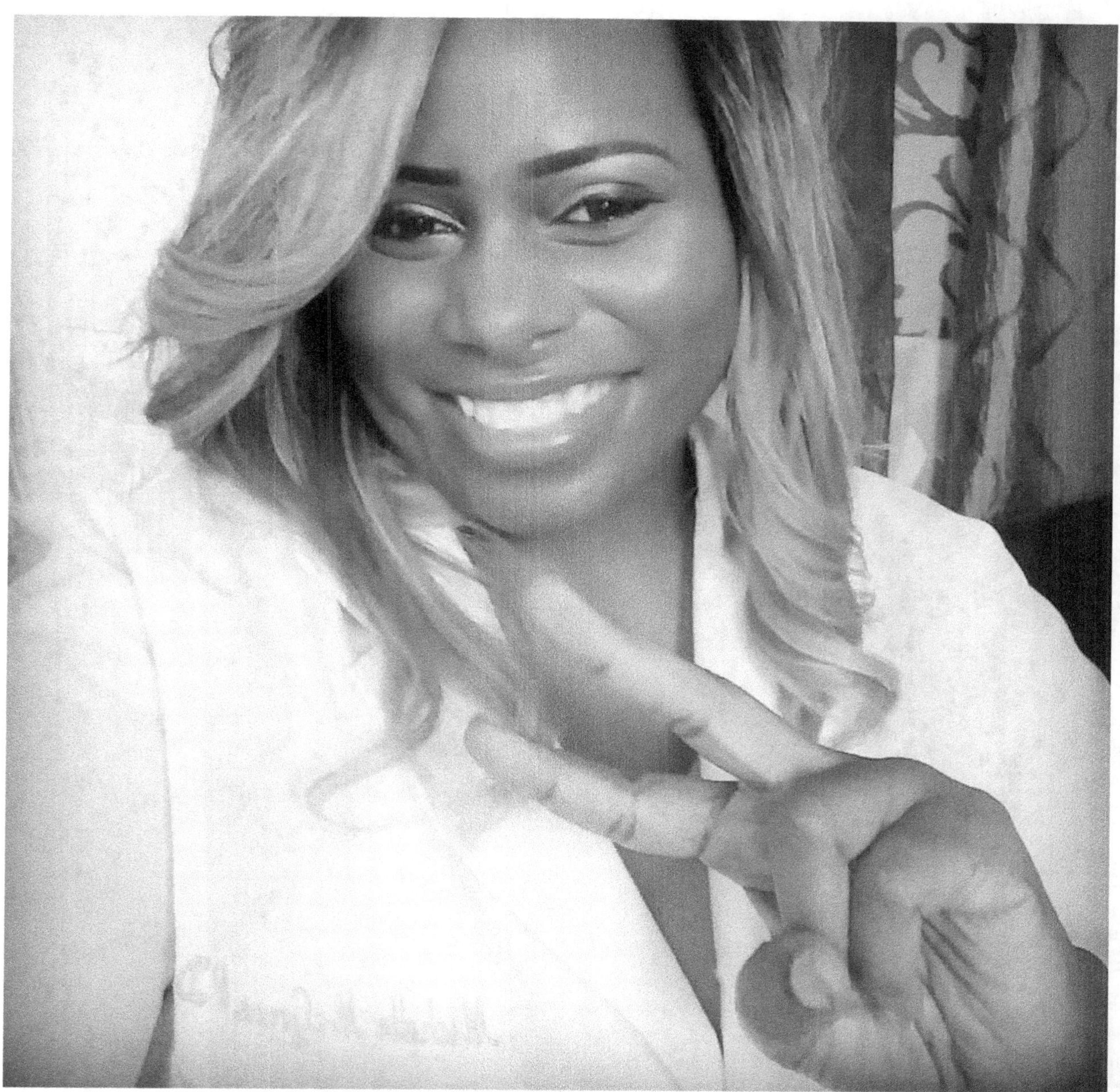

I began feeling numbness and tingling in fingers and

joints.

Back

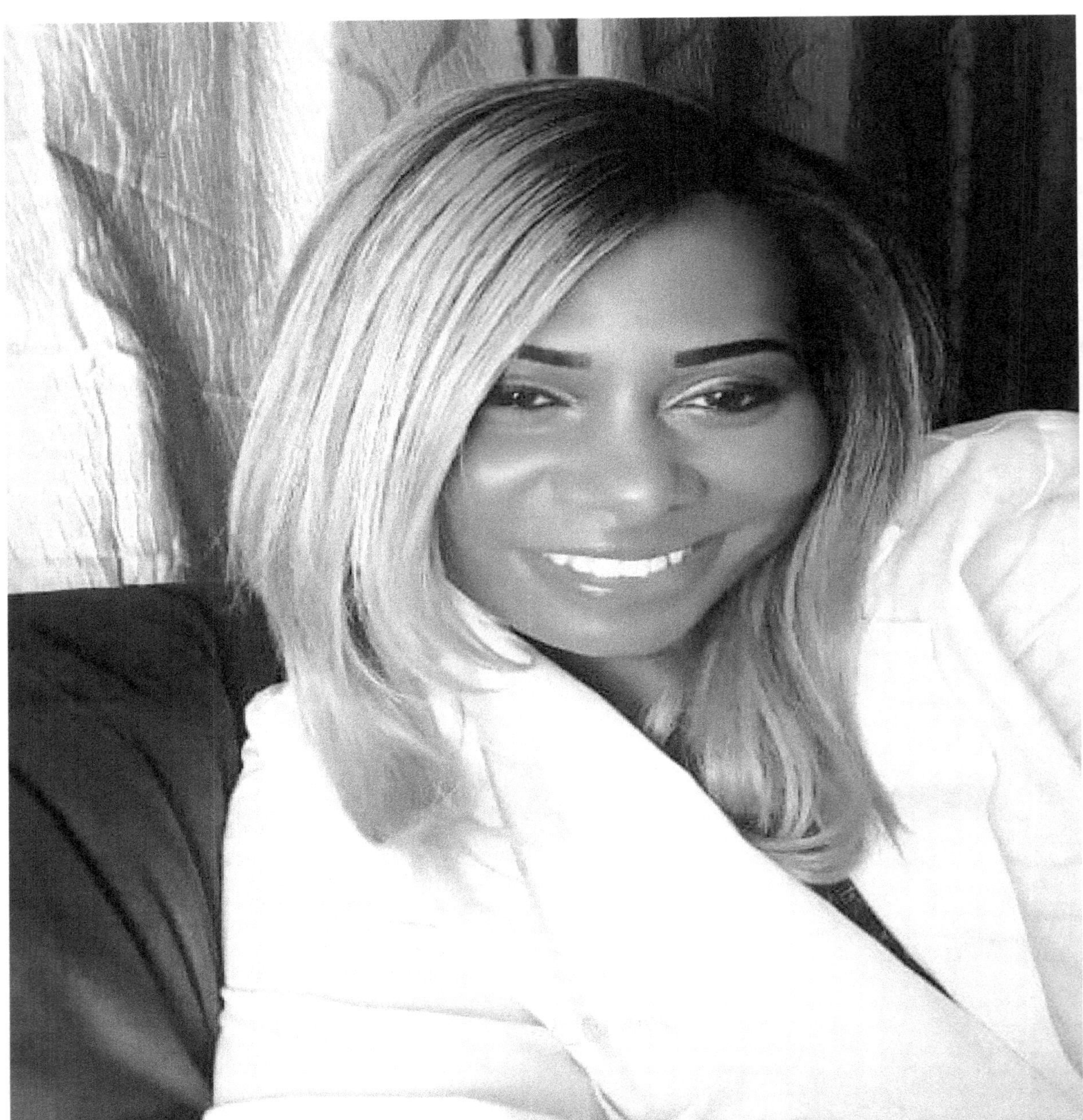

My lower back began aching.

Knees

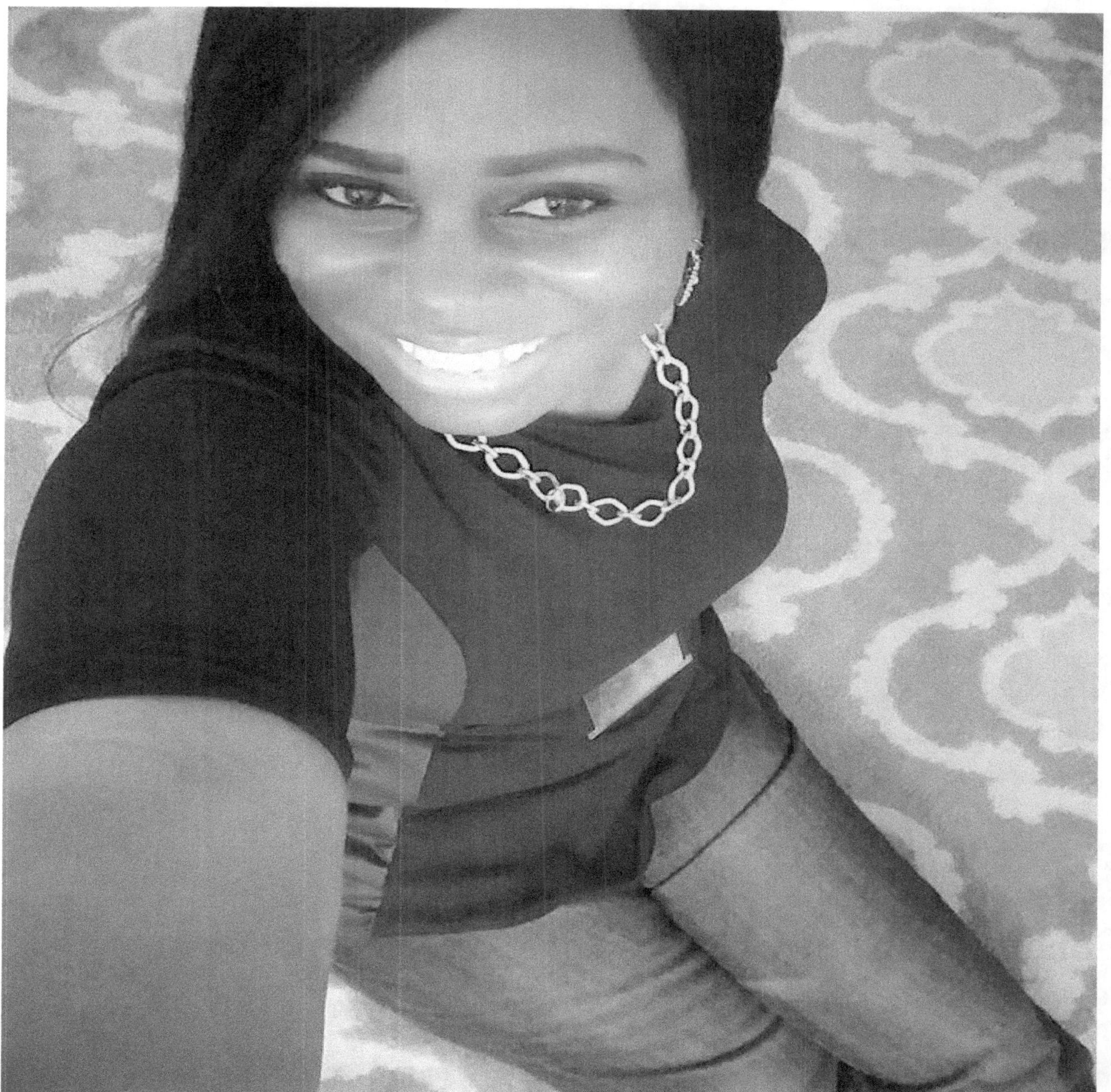

I could feel my knees begin to ache during the day

without agitation.

Feet

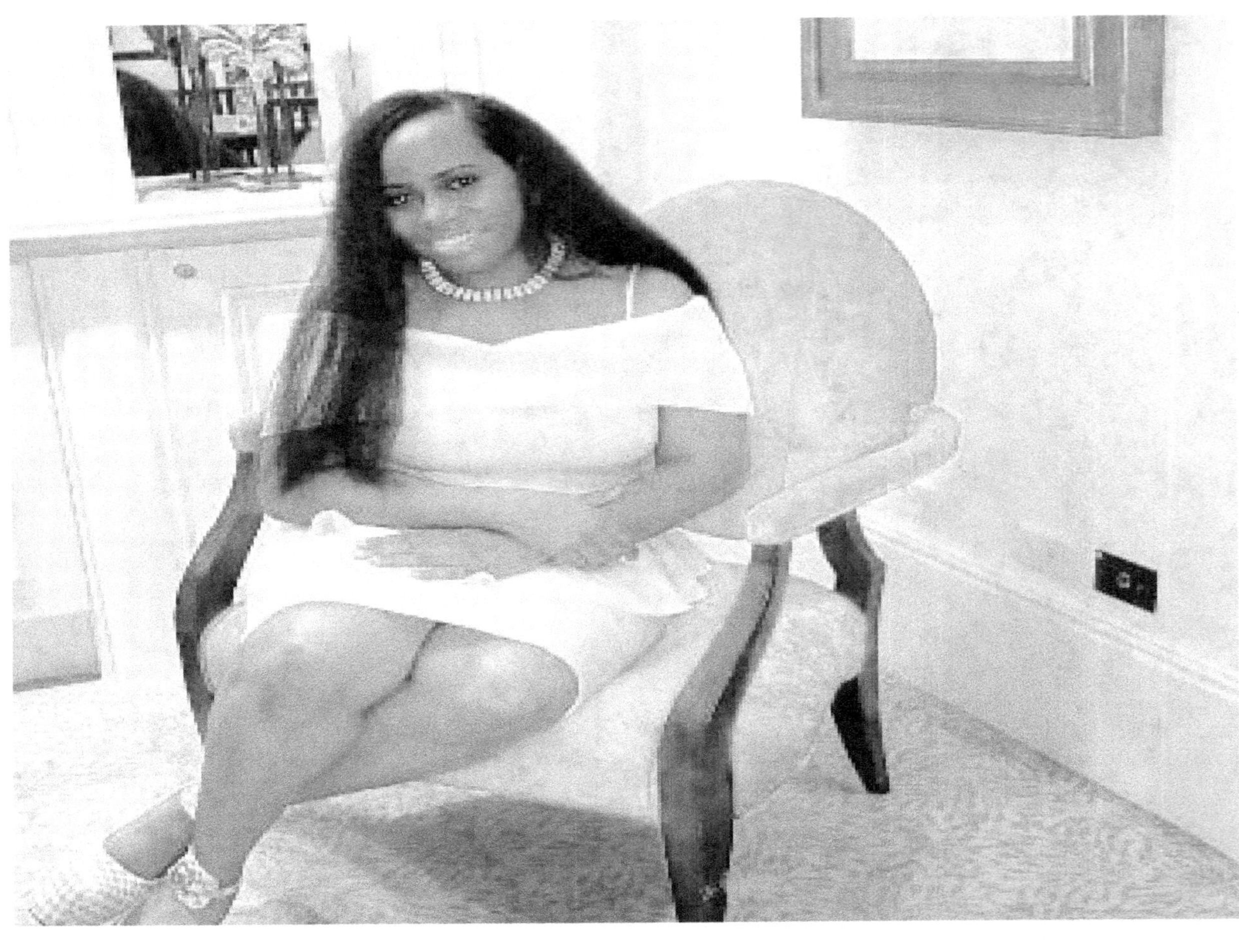

I noticed that my feet and ankles were swollen.

Internal Organs

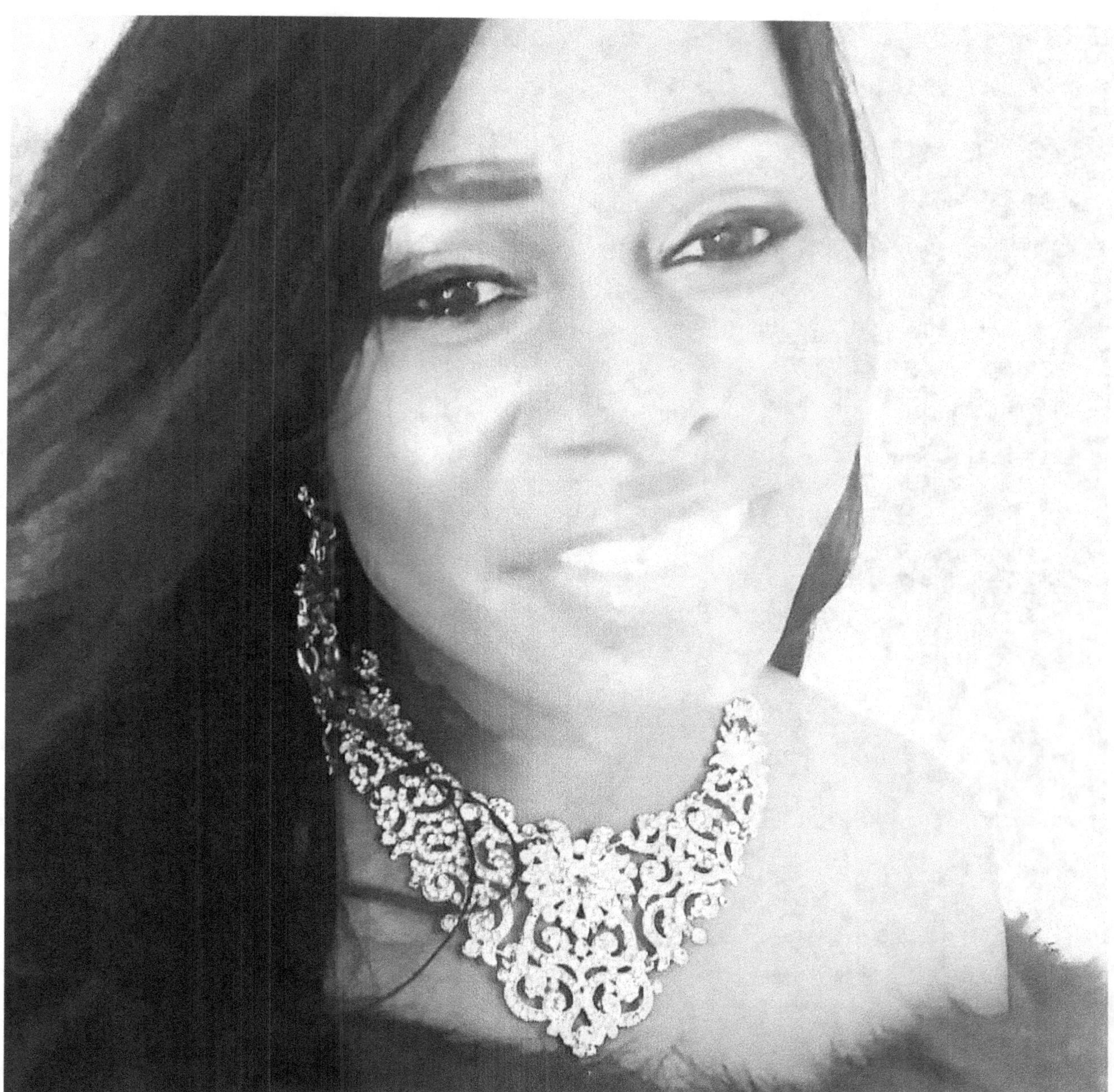

My internal organs begin to hurt. I could even feel my

kidneys aching.

Overall Feeling

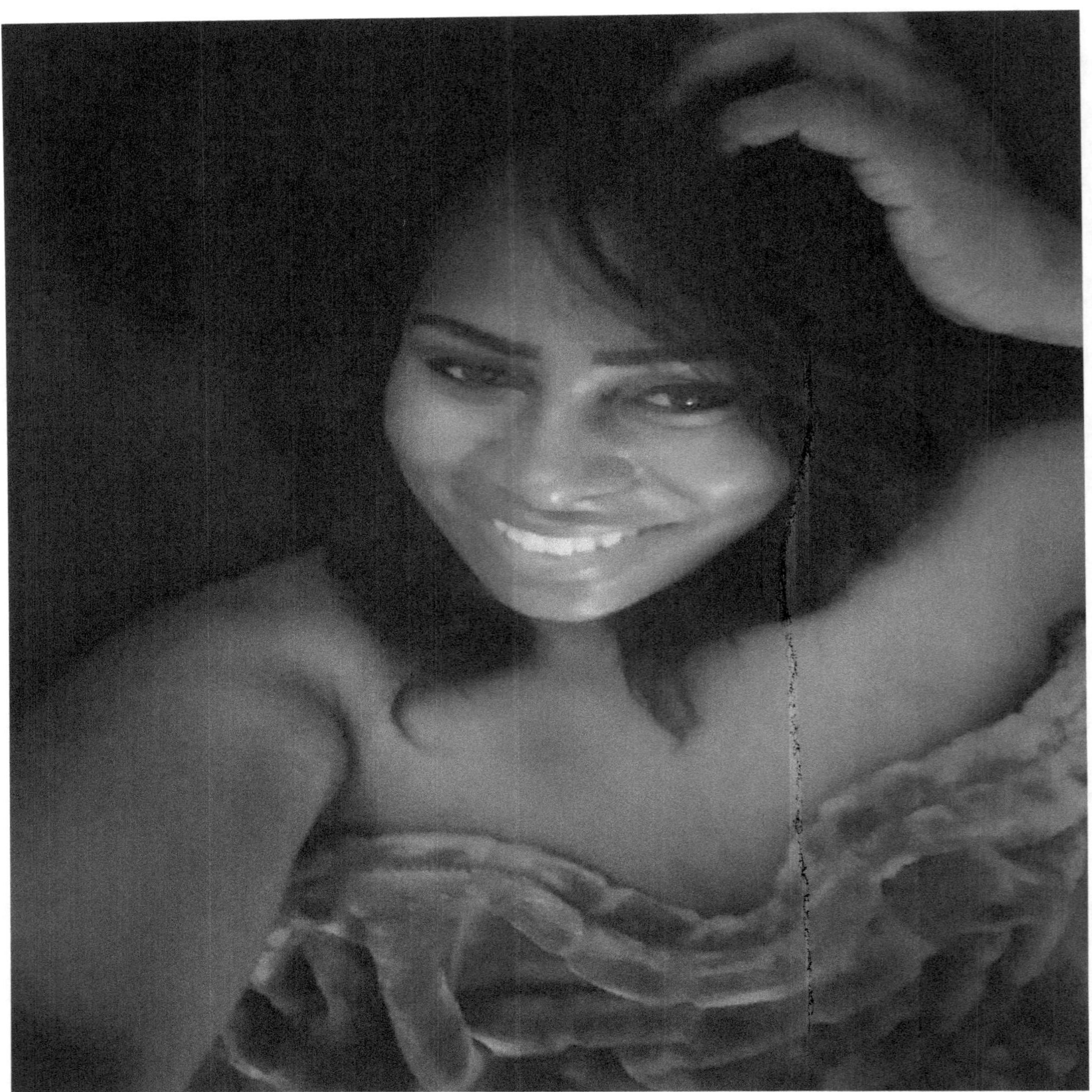

During this time, overall I felt just awful. I gained almost

thirty pounds. The feeling of being sluggish all the time

and burnt out I believe was the worst for me because I

was too exhausted to do anything else. Sometimes, I felt

a little light-headed and dizzy having to catch myself. I

began sweating more and had to switch up on deodorants.

Solutions

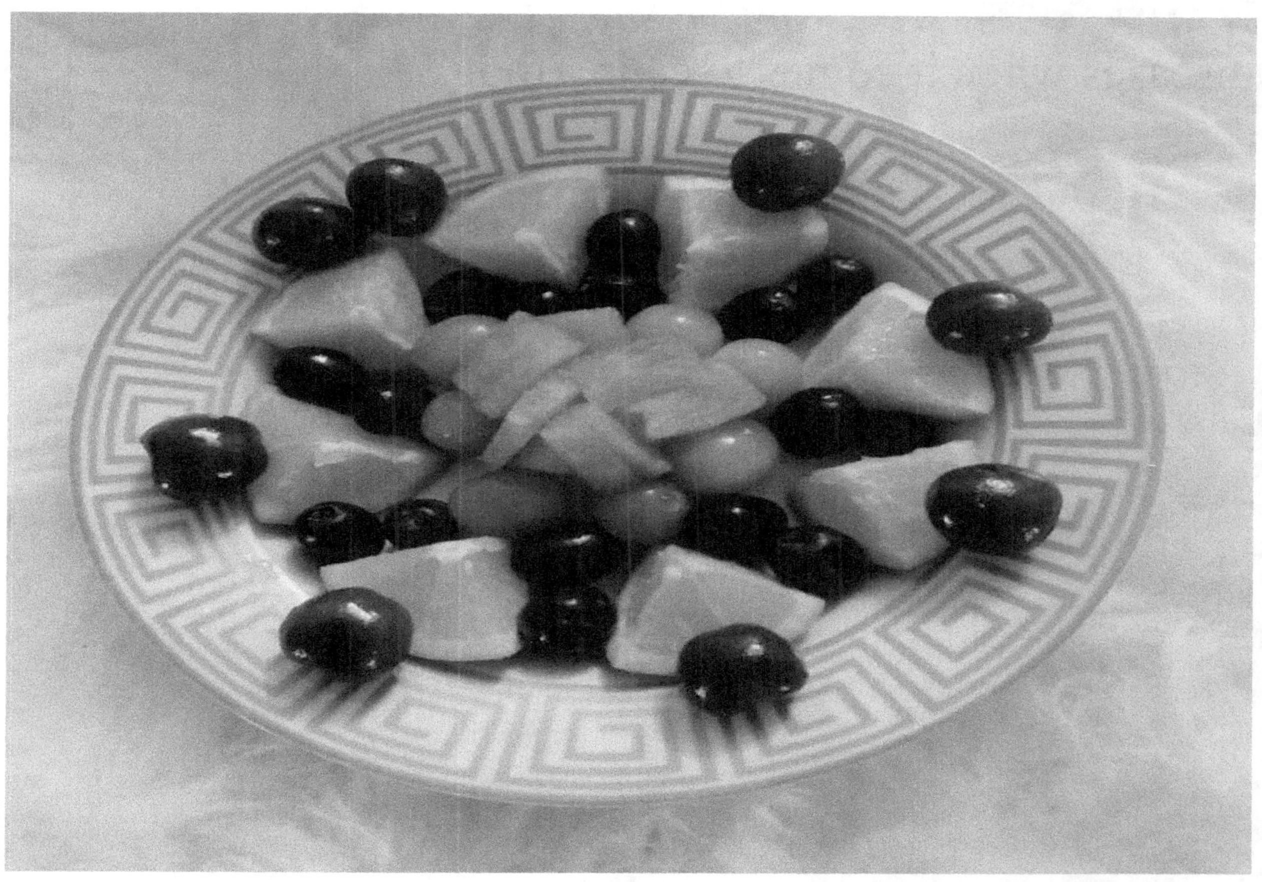

My solutions are simply. For me to rectify all of the

issues that I have created by eating a diet that lack life, I

will consume foods with light (will be in another book),

detox, and fast. It is just that simple. I could also

incorporate a daily exercise regimen to speed up the

process. The next book will talk about the discovery of

this one thing the plagues human with ailments and

diseases when it comes to eating food.